The Keto Vegetarian Lifestyle

Lose Weight & be Healthy

with Yummy Vegetarian Recipes

Ricardo Abagnale

0

by reading this document, the reader agrees that under no circumstances is the author responsible for any losses, direct or indirect, which are incurred as a result of the use of information contained within this document, including, but not limited to, — errors, omissions, or inaccuracies.

Table of Contents

INTRODUCTION 6

BREAKFAST 7

   HEALTHY KETO PANCAKES 7

   KETO PROTEIN BREAKFAST MUFFINS 9

MAINS 11

   CINNAMON CAULIFLOWER RICE, ZUCCHINIS AND SPINACH 11

   ASPARAGUS, BOK CHOY AND RADISH MIX 13

   KALE AND CUCUMBER SALAD 15

   AVOCADO, ENDIVE AND ASPARAGUS MIX 17

   BELL PEPPERS AND SPINACH PAN 19

   MUSHROOMS AND ASPARAGUS MIX 21

   KALE AND RAISINS...23

   COLLARD GREENS AND GARLIC MIX 25

   VEGGIE HASH 27

SIDES...29

   GINGER MUSHROOMS...29

   BELL PEPPER SAUTÉ 31

   KALE AND TOMATOES 33

   CHILI ARTICHOKES..35

   BRUSSELS SPROUTS MIX..37

   CAULIFLOWER MIX...39

FRUIT AND VEGETABLES 41

   EGGPLANT HASH 41

   EGGPLANT JAM...43

   WARM WATERCRESS MIX...45

   WATERCRESS SOUP..47

ARTICHOKES AND MUSHROOM MIX 49

SOUPS AND STEWS **52**

SQUASH SOUP WITH PECANS AND GINGER.....................................52

ROOT VEGETABLE BISQUE 54

CURRIED PUMPKIN SOUP 56

KETO PASTA **58**

TOFU AND SPINACH LASAGNA WITH RED SAUCE...........................58

ZOODLE BOLOGNESE 63

SALADS **66**

INDONESIAN GREEN BEAN SALAD WITH CABBAGE AND CARROTS 66

CUCUMBER AND ONION QUINOA SALAD 68

MOROCCAN AUBERGINE SALAD 70

POTATO SALAD WITH ARTICHOKE HEARTS 73

SNACKS **75**

CAPERS DIP 75

RADISH AND WALNUTS DIP 77

MUSHROOM CAKES 79

CABBAGE STICKS 81

CRISPY BRUSSELS SPROUTS 83

DESSERTS **85**

COCONUT CHOCOLATE CAKE 85

MINT CHOCOLATE CREAM 87

CRANBERRIES CAKE 89

SWEET ZUCCHINI BUNS 91

LIME CUSTARD 93

WARM RUM BUTTER SPICED CIDER 95

PEPPERMINT PATTY COCOA 96

APPLE & WALNUT CAKE 97

OTHER RECIPES **99**

LEMON GARLIC MUSHROOMS.. 99

ALMOND GREEN BEANS.. 101

FRIED OKRA 103

TOMATO AVOCADO CUCUMBER SALAD......................................105

ASIAN CUCUMBER SALAD... 107

ROASTED CARROTS 109

INTRODUCTION

The Ketogenic diet is truly life changing. The diet improves your overall health and helps you lose the extra weight in a matter of days. The diet will show its multiple benefits even from the beginning and it will become your new lifestyle really soon.

As soon as you embrace the Ketogenic diet, you will start to live a completely new life.

On the other hand, the vegetarian diet is such a healthy dietary option you can choose when trying to live healthy and also lose some weight.

The collection we bring to you today is actually a combination between the Ketogenic and vegetarian diets. You get to discover some amazing Ketogenic vegetarian dishes you can prepare in the comfort of your own home.

All the dishes you found here follow both the Ketogenic and the vegetarian rules, they all taste delicious and rich and they are all easy to make.

We can assure you that such a combo is hard to find. So, start a keto diet with a vegetarian "touch" today. It will be both useful and fun!

So, what are you still waiting for? Get started with the Ketogenic diet and learn how to prepare the best and most flavored Ketogenic vegetarian dishes. Enjoy them all!

Healthy Keto Pancakes

Preparation time: 10 minutes

Cooking time: 2 minutes

Servings: 6

Ingredients:

- 1 large banana, mashed
- 2 organic eggs
- 1/8 teaspoon baking powder
- tablespoons vanilla protein powder

Nutritional Values (Per Serving):

- Calories: 78
- Fat: 1.6 g
- Carbohydrates: 5.5 g
- Sugar: 3 g
- Protein: 11.1 g
- Cholesterol: 55 mg

Directions:

1. Heat your pan over medium heat.
2. In a mixing bowl add all your ingredients and mix well to combine.
3. Spray pan with cooking spray. Pour 3 tablespoons of batter into the hot pan to make the pancake. Cook the pancake for no more than 1 minute and flip onto other side and cook for an additional minute.
4. Serve with sugar-free syrup. Enjoy!

Keto Protein Breakfast Muffins

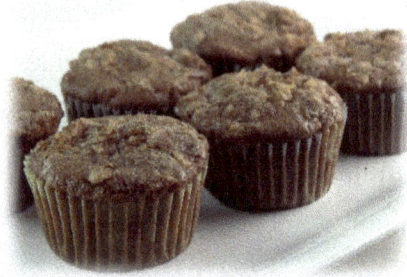

Preparation time: 12 minutes

Cooking time: 25 minutes

Servings: 12

Nutritional Values (Per Serving): (Per Serving):

- Calories: 148
- Fat: 12.3 g
- Carbohydrates: 2 g
- Sugar: 0.4 g
- Protein: 7.8 g
- Cholesterol: 116 mg

Ingredients:

- 8 organic eggs
- 8-ounces cream cheese

- 4 tablespoons butter, melted
- 2 scoops protein powder

Directions:

1. Mix cream cheese and melted butter in a mixing bowl. Add eggs and protein powder and mix well.
2. With the use of a hand mixer mix until well combined and spray your muffin pan with cooking spray.
3. Fill each muffin cup ¾ full of mixture.
4. Bake for 25 minutes in preheated oven at 350°Fahrenheit.
5. Serve and enjoy!

Cinnamon Cauliflower Rice, Zucchinis and Spinach

Preparation time: 10 minutes

Cooking time: 10 minutes

Servings: 4

Nutritional Values (Per Serving):

- Calories 189
- Fat 2
- Fiber 2
- Carbs 20
- Protein 7

Ingredients:

- 1 cup cauliflower rice

- 2 tablespoons olive oil 1 zucchini, sliced
- 1 cup baby spinach
- ½ cup veggie stock
- ½ teaspoon turmeric powder
- ¼ teaspoon cinnamon powder
- A pinch of sea salt and black pepper
- 1/3 cup dates, dried and chopped
- 1 tablespoon almonds, chopped
- ¼ cup chives, chopped

Directions:

1. Heat up a pan with the oil over medium heat, add the cauliflower rice, dates, turmeric and cinnamon and sauté for 3 minutes.
2. Add the zucchini and the other ingredients, toss, cook the mix for 7 minutes more, divide between plates and serve.

Asparagus, Bok Choy and Radish Mix

Preparation time: 10 minutes

Cooking time: 12 minutes

Servings: 4

Nutritional Values (Per Serving):

- Calories 140
- Fat 1
- Fiber 10
- Carbs 20
- Protein 8

Ingredients:

- ½ pound asparagus, trimmed and halved
- 1 cup bok choy, torn
- 1 cup radishes, halved

- 2 tablespoons balsamic vinegar
- 2 tablespoons olive oil
- 2 teaspoon Italian seasoning
- 2 teaspoons garlic powder
- 1 teaspoon coriander, ground
- 1 teaspoon fennel seeds, crushed
- 1 tablespoon chives, chopped

Directions:

1. Heat up a pan with the oil over medium heat, add the asparagus, bok choy, the radishes and the other ingredients, toss, cook for 12 minutes, divide between plates and serve.

Kale and Cucumber Salad

Preparation time: 10 minutes

Cooking time: 0 minutes

Servings: 4

Nutritional Values (Per Serving):

- Calories 90
- Fat 1
- Fiber 3
- Carbs 7
- Protein 2

Ingredients:

- 2 cups baby kale
- 2 cucumbers, sliced
- 2 tablespoons avocado oil
- 1 cup coconut cream

- 1 teaspoon balsamic vinegar
- 2 tablespoons dill, chopped

Directions:

1. In a bowl, combine the kale with the cucumbers and the other ingredients, toss and serve.

Avocado, Endive and Asparagus Mix

Preparation time: 10 minutes

Cooking time: 10 minutes

Servings: 4

Nutritional Values (Per Serving):

- Calories 111
- Fat 2
- Fiber 5
- Carbs 8
- Protein 2

Ingredients:

- 2 avocados, peeled, pitted and sliced
- 2 endives, shredded
- 4 asparagus spears, trimmed and halved

- 2 tablespoons sesame seeds
- 2 tablespoons avocado oil
- Juice of 1 lime
- A pinch of sea salt and black pepper
- Black pepper to the taste
- 1 tablespoon chives, chopped

Directions:

1. Heat up a pan with the oil over medium heat, add the endives, asparagus, avocados and the other ingredients, toss, cook for 10 minutes, divide between plates and serve.

Bell Peppers and Spinach Pan

Preparation time: 10 minutes

Cooking time: 12 minutes

Servings: 4

Nutritional Values (Per Serving):

- Calories 125
- Fat 3
- Fiber 5
- Carbs 9
- Protein 12

Ingredients:

- 1 tablespoon olive oil
- 1 red bell pepper, cut into strips
- 1 green bell pepper, cut into strips
- 1 orange bell pepper, cut into strips
- 2 cups baby spinach

- 3 garlic cloves, minced
- 2 teaspoons garlic powder
- A pinch of sea salt and black pepper
- 1 teaspoon fennel seeds, crushed
- 1 teaspoon chili powder

Directions:

1. Heat up a pan with the oil over medium high heat, add the peppers and the garlic and sauté for 2 minutes.
2. Add the spinach and the other ingredients, toss, cook over medium heat for 10 minutes more, divide between plates and serve.

Mushrooms and Asparagus Mix

Preparation time: 10 minutes

Cooking time: 15 minutes

Servings: 4

Nutritional Values (Per Serving):

- Calories 74
- Fat 4.6
- Fiber 2.6
- Carbs 6.9
- Protein 4.7

Ingredients:

- 1 pound white mushrooms, sliced
- 1 asparagus bunch, trimmed and halved
- 1 teaspoon sweet paprika
- 1 teaspoon coriander, ground
- 1 teaspoon chili powder

- ½ teaspoon thyme, dried
- 2 garlic cloves, minced
- ¼ cup coconut cream
- 1 tablespoon avocado oil

Directions:

1. Heat up a pan with the oil over medium high heat, add the mushrooms, the asparagus and the other ingredients, toss, cook for 15 minutes, divide between plates and serve.

Kale and Raisins

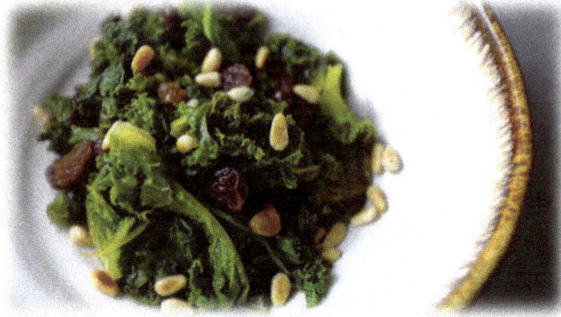

Preparation time: 10 minutes

Cooking time: 20 minutes

Servings: 4

Nutritional Values (Per Serving):

- Calories 102
- Fat 1.2
- Fiber 2.7
- Carbs 21.4
- Protein 4

Ingredients:

- 1 pound kale, torn
- 1 tomato, cubed
- 2 tablespoons avocado oil
- Juice of 1 lime
- ¼ cup raisins
- 1 teaspoon nutmeg, ground
- ½ teaspoon ginger, grated
- ½ teaspoon cinnamon powder
- 1 tablespoon chives, chopped
- A pinch of sea salt and black pepper

Directions:

1. Heat up a pan with the oil over medium heat, add the kale, tomato, lime juice and the other ingredients, toss, cook for 20 minutes, divide into bowls and serve.

Collard Greens and Garlic Mix

Preparation time: 10 minutes

Cooking time: 10 minutes

Servings: 4

Nutritional Values (Per Serving):

- Calories 130
- Fat 1
- Fiber 8
- Carbs 10
- Protein 6

Ingredients:

- 2 tablespoons avocado oil
- 4 garlic cloves, minced
- 4 bunches collard greens
- 1 tomato, cubed
- A pinch of sea salt and black pepper

- Black pepper to the taste
- 1 tablespoon almonds, chopped

Directions:

1. Heat up a pan with the oil over medium heat, add the garlic, collard greens and the other ingredients, toss well, cook for 10 minutes, divide into bowls and serve.

Veggie Hash

Preparation time: 10 minutes

Cooking time: 20 minutes

Servings: 4

Nutritional Values (Per Serving):

- Calories 135
- Fat 2
- Fiber 4
- Carbs 5.4
- Protein 5

Ingredients:

- 1 bunch asparagus, chopped
- 2 cups radishes, halved
- ½ cup mushrooms, halved
- 3 tablespoons olive oil
- 1 shallot, chopped

- ½ cup roasted bell peppers, chopped
- 2 garlic cloves, minced
- A pinch of salt and black pepper
- 1 tablespoon chives, chopped
- 1 tablespoon sage, chopped

Directions:

1. Heat up a pan with the oil over medium heat, add the shallot and the garlic and sauté for 5 minutes.
2. Add the mushrooms and sauté for 5 minutes more.
3. Add the rest of the ingredients, toss, cook everything over medium heat for another 10 minutes, divide into bowls and serve.

Ginger Mushrooms

Preparation time: 10 minutes

Cooking time: 20 minutes

Servings: 4

Nutritional Values (Per Serving):

- Calories 120
- Fat 2
- Fiber 2
- Carbs 4
- Protein 5

Ingredients:

- 1 pound mushrooms, sliced
- 1 yellow onion, chopped
- 1 tablespoon ginger, grated

- 1 tablespoon olive oil
- 2 tablespoons balsamic vinegar
- 2 garlic cloves, minced
- A pinch of salt and black pepper
- ¼ cup lime juice
- 2 tablespoons walnuts, chopped

Directions:

1. Heat up a pan with the oil over medium-high heat, add the onion and the ginger and sauté for 5 minutes.
2. Add the mushrooms and the other ingredients, toss, cook over medium heat for 15 minutes more, divide between plates and serve.

Bell Pepper Sauté

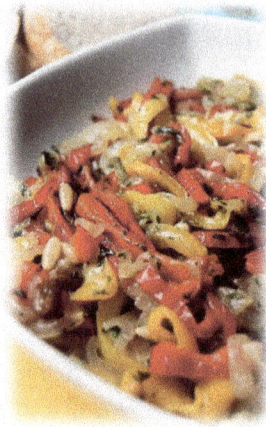

Preparation time: 5 minutes

Cooking time: 20 minutes

Servings: 4

Nutritional Values (Per Serving):

- Calories 120
- Fat 1
- Fiber 2
- Carbs 7
- Protein 6

Ingredients:

- 1 red bell pepper, cut into strips
- 1 yellow bell pepper, cut into strips
- 1 green bell pepper, cut into strips
- 1 orange bell pepper, cut into strips
- 3 scallions, chopped
- 1 tablespoon olive oil
- 1 tablespoon coconut aminos
- A pinch of salt and black pepper
- 1 tablespoon parsley, chopped
- 1 tablespoon rosemary, chopped

Directions:

1. Heat up a pan with the oil over medium-high heat, add the scallions and sauté for 5 minutes.
2. Add the bell peppers and the other ingredients, toss, cook over medium heat for 15 minutes more, divide between plates and serve.

Kale and Tomatoes

Preparation time: 5 minutes

Cooking time: 20 minutes

Servings: 4

Nutritional Values (Per Serving):

- Calories 170
- Fat 6
- Fiber 6
- Carbs 9
- Protein 4

Ingredients:

- 1 cup cherry tomatoes, halved
- 1 pound baby kale
- 1 yellow onion, chopped
- 2 tablespoons olive oil
- 1 tablespoon balsamic vinegar

- 1 tablespoon cilantro, chopped
- 2 tablespoons vegetable stock
- A pinch of salt and black pepper

Directions:

1. Heat up a pan with the oil over medium heat, add the onion and sauté for 5 minutes.
2. Add the kale, tomatoes and the other ingredients, toss, cook over medium heat for 15 minutes more, divide between plates and serve as a side dish.

Chili Artichokes

Preparation time: 10 minutes

Cooking time: 25 minutes

Servings: 4

Nutritional Values (Per Serving):

- Calories 132
- Fat 2
- Fiber 2
- Carbs 4
- Protein 6

Ingredients:

- 2 artichokes, trimmed and halved
- 1 teaspoon chili powder
- 2 green chilies, mined
- 2 tablespoons olive oil
- 1 teaspoon garlic powder

- 1 teaspoon sweet paprika
- A pinch of salt and black pepper
- Juice of 1 lime

Directions:

1. In a roasting pan, combine the artichokes with the chili powder, the chilies and the other ingredients, toss and bake at 380 degrees F for 25 minutes.
2. Divide the artichokes between plates and serve.

Brussels Sprouts Mix

Preparation time: 10 minutes

Cooking time: 20 minutes

Servings: 4

Nutritional Values (Per Serving):

- Calories 160
- Fat 2
- Fiber 2
- Carbs 4
- Protein 5

Ingredients:

- 2 tablespoons olive oil
- 1 pound Brussels sprouts, trimmed and halved
- 1 tablespoon ginger, grated
- 2 garlic cloves, minced

- 1 tablespoon pine nuts
- 1 tablespoon olive oil

Directions:

1. Heat up a pan with the oil over medium heat, add the garlic and the ginger and sauté for 2 minutes.
2. Add the Brussels sprouts and the other ingredients, toss, cook for 18 minutes more, divide between plates and serve.

Cauliflower Mix

Preparation time: 10 minutes

Cooking time: 25 minutes

Servings: 4

Nutritional Values (Per Serving):

- Calories 160
- Fat 3
- Fiber 2
- Carbs 9
- Protein 4

Ingredients:

- 1 pound cauliflower florets
- 2 tablespoons avocado oil
- 1 teaspoon nutmeg, ground
- 1 teaspoon hot paprika
- 1 tablespoon pumpkin seeds

- 1 tablespoon chives, chopped
- A pinch of sea salt and black pepper

Directions:

1. Spread the cauliflower florets on a baking sheet lined with parchment paper, add the oil, the nutmeg and the other ingredients, toss and bake at 380 degrees F for 25 minutes.
2. Divide the cauliflower mix between plates and serve as a side dish.

Eggplant Hash

Preparation time: 20 minutes

Cooking time: 20 minutes

Servings: 4

Nutritional Values (Per Serving):

- calories 258
- fat 25,6
- fiber 5,1
- carbs 9,5
- protein 1.9

Ingredients:

- 1 eggplant, roughly chopped
- ½ cup olive oil
- ½ pound cherry tomatoes, halved

- 1 teaspoon Tabasco sauce
- ¼ cup basil, chopped
- ¼ cup mint, chopped
- A pinch of sea salt Black pepper to taste

Directions:

1. Put eggplant pieces in a bowl, add a pinch of salt, toss to coat, leave aside for 20 minutes and drain using paper towels.
2. Heat up a pan with half of the oil over medium-high heat, add eggplant, cook for 3 minutes, flip, cook them for 3 minutes more and transfer to a bowl.
3. Heat up the same pan with the rest of the oil over medium-high heat, add tomatoes and cook them for 8 minutes stirring from time to time.
4. Return eggplant pieces to the pan and add a pinch of salt, black pepper, basil, mint and Tabasco sauce.
5. Stir, cook for 2 minutes more, divide between plates and serve.
6. Enjoy!

Eggplant Jam

Preparation time: 10 minutes

Cooking time: 1 hour

Servings: 6

Nutritional Values (Per Serving):

- Calories 75
- Fat 0,7
- Fiber 10,1
- Carbs 17,2
- Protein 3

Ingredients:

- 3 eggplants, sliced lengthwise
- 2 teaspoons sweet paprika
- 2 garlic cloves, minced
- A pinch of sea salt
- A pinch of cinnamon, ground

- 1 teaspoon cumin, ground
- A splash of hot sauce
- ¼ cup water
- 1 tablespoon parsley, chopped
- 2 tablespoons lemon juice

Directions:

1. Sprinkle some salt on eggplant slices and leave them aside for 10 minutes.
2. Pat dry eggplant, brush them with half of the oil, place on a lined baking sheet, place in the oven at 375 degrees F, bake for 25 minutes flipping them halfway and leave them aside to cool down.
3. In a bowl, mix paprika with garlic, cinnamon, cumin, water and hot sauce and stir well.
4. Add baked eggplant pieces and mash them with a fork.
5. Heat up a pan with the rest of the oil over medium-low heat, add eggplant mix, stir and cook for 20 minutes.
6. Add lemon juice and parsley, stir, take off heat, divide into small bowls and serve.
7. Enjoy!

Warm Watercress Mix

Preparation time: 10 minutes

Cooking time: 10 minutes

Servings: 4

Nutritional Values (Per Serving):

- Calories 220
- Fat 21,8
- Fiber 2,1
- Carbs 2,9
- Protein 5,3

Ingredients:

- 1 pound watercress, chopped
- ¼ cup olive oil
- 1 garlic clove, cut in halves
- 1 small shallot, peeled, cooked and chopped
- ¼ cup hazelnuts, chopped

- Black pepper to taste
- ¼ cup pine nuts

Directions:

1. Heat up a pan with the oil over medium heat, add garlic clove halves, cook for 2 minutes and discard.
2. Heat up the pan with the garlic oil again over medium heat, add hazelnuts and pine nuts, stir and cook for 6 minutes.
3. Add shallots, black pepper to taste and watercress, stir, cook for 2 minutes, divide between plates and serve right away.
4. Enjoy!

Watercress Soup

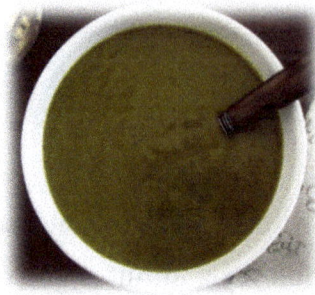

Preparation time: 10 minutes

Cooking time: 20 minutes

Servings: 4

Nutritional Values (Per Serving):

- Calories 224
- Fat 11,8
- Fiber 5,7
- Carbs 29,6
- Protein 4

Ingredients:

- 8 ounces watercress
- 1 tablespoon lemon juice
- A pinch of nutmeg, ground
- 4 ounces coconut milk
- A pinch of sea salt Black pepper to taste
- 14 ounces veggie stock
- 1 celery stick, chopped
- 1 onion, chopped
- 1 tablespoon olive oil
- 12 ounces sweet potatoes, peeled and chopped

Directions:

1. Heat up a large saucepan with the oil over medium heat, add onion and celery, stir and cook for 5 minutes.
2. Add sweet potato pieces and stock, stir, bring to a simmer, cover and cook on a low heat for 10 minutes.
3. Add watercress, stir, cover saucepan again and cook for 5 minutes.
4. Blend this with an immersion blender, add a pinch of nutmeg, lemon juice, salt, pepper and coconut milk, bring to a simmer again, divide into bowls and serve.
5. Enjoy!

Artichokes and Mushroom Mix

Preparation time: 30 minutes

Cooking time: 30 minutes

Servings: 4

Nutritional Values (Per Serving):

- Calories 354
- Fat 29,9
- Fiber 4,3
- Carbs 16,5
- Protein 6,6

Ingredients:

- 16 mushrooms, sliced
- 1/3 cup tamari sauce
- 1/3 cup olive oil
- 4 tablespoons balsamic vinegar
- 4 garlic cloves, minced

- 1 tablespoon lemon juice
- 1 teaspoon oregano, dried
- 1 teaspoon rosemary, dried
- ½ tablespoon thyme, dried
- A pinch of sea salt
- Black pepper to taste
- 1 sweet onion, chopped
- 1 jar artichoke hearts
- 4 cups spinach
- 1 tablespoon coconut oil
- 1 teaspoon garlic, minced
- 1 cauliflower head, florets separated
- ½ cup veggie stock
- 1 teaspoon garlic powder
- A pinch of nutmeg, ground

Directions:

1. In a bowl, mix vinegar with tamari sauce, lemon juice, 4 garlic cloves, olive oil, oregano, rosemary, thyme, a pinch of salt, black pepper and mushrooms, toss to coat well and leave aside for 30 minutes.

2. Transfer these to a lined baking sheet and bake them in the oven at 350 degrees F for 30 minutes.

3. In a food processor, mix cauliflower with a pinch of sea salt and black pepper and pulse until you obtain rice.

4. Heat a pan to medium-high heat, add cauliflower rice, toast for 2 minutes, add nutmeg, garlic powder, black pepper and stock, stir and cook until stock evaporated.

5. Heat a pan with the coconut oil over medium heat, add onion, artichokes, 1 teaspoon garlic and spinach, stir and cook for a few minutes.

6. Divide cauliflower rice on plates, top with artichokes and mushrooms and serve.

Squash Soup with Pecans and Ginger

Preparation time: 10 minutes

Cooking time: 30 minutes

Servings: 4

Ingredients:

- 1/3 cup toasted pecans
- 2 tablespoons chopped crystallized ginger
- 1 tablespoon canola or grapeseed oil
- 1 medium onion, chopped
- 1 celery rib, chopped
- 1 teaspoon grated fresh ginger
- 5 cups vegetable broth (homemade, store-bought or water)
- 1 kabocha squash, peeled, seeded, and cut into 1/2-inch dice

- ¼ cup pure maple syrup
- 2 tablespoons soy sauce
- ¼ teaspoon ground allspice
- Salt and freshly ground black pepper
- 1 cup plain unsweetened soy milk

Directions:

1. In a food processor, combine the pecans and crystallized ginger and pulse until coarsely chopped. Set aside.
2. In a large soup pot, heat the oil over medium heat. Add the onion, celery, and fresh ginger. Cover and cook until softened, about 5 minutes. Stir in the broth and squash, cover, and bring to a boil. Reduce the heat to low and simmer, covered, stirring occasionally, until the squash is tender, about 30 minutes.
3. Stir in the maple syrup, soy sauce, allspice, and salt and pepper to taste. Puree in the pot with an immersion blender or in a blender or food processor, in batches if necessary, and return to the pot.
4. Stir in the soy milk and heat over low heat until hot. Ladle the soup into bowls and sprinkle with the pecan and ginger mixture, and serve.

Root Vegetable Bisque

Preparation time: 5 minutes

Cooking time: 35 minutes

Servings: 4 to 6

Ingredients:

- 1 tablespoon olive oil
- 3 large shallots, chopped
- 2 large carrots, shredded
- 2 medium parsnips, shredded
- 1 medium potato, peeled and chopped
- 2 garlic cloves, minced
- 1/2 teaspoon dried thyme
- 1/4 teaspoon dried marjoram
- 4 cups vegetable broth (homemade, store-bought or water)
- 1 cup plain unsweetened soy milk
- Salt and freshly ground black pepper
- 1 tablespoon minced fresh parsley, garnish

Directions:

1. In a large soup pot, heat the oil over medium heat. Add the shallots, carrots, parsnips, potato, and garlic. Cover and cook until softened, about 5 minutes. Add the thyme, marjoram, and broth and bring to a boil. Reduce heat to low and simmer, uncovered, until the vegetables are tender, about 30 minutes.

2. Puree the soup in the pot with an immersion blender or in a blender or food processor in batches if necessary, then return to the pot. Stir in the soy milk and taste, adjusting seasonings if necessary. Heat the soup over low heat until hot. Ladle into bowls, sprinkle with parsley, and serve.

Curried Pumpkin Soup

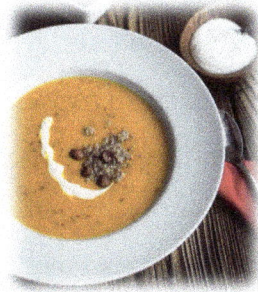

Preparation time: 5 minutes

Cooking time: 22 minutes

Servings: 4 to 6

Ingredients:

- 1 tablespoon olive oil
- 1 medium onion, chopped
- 1 garlic clove, minced
- 1 teaspoon grated fresh ginger
- 1 tablespoon hot or mild curry powder
- 1 16-ouncecan pumpkin puree or 2 cups cooked fresh pumpkin
- 3 cups vegetable broth (homemade, store-bought or water)

- Salt
- 1 13.5-ouncecan unsweetened coconut milk
- 1 tablespoon minced fresh parsley, for garnish
- Mango chutney, for garnish (optional)
- Chopped roasted cashews, for garnish (optional)

Directions:

1. In a large soup pot, heat the oil over medium heat. Add the onion and garlic and cover and cook until softened, about 7 minutes. Stir in the ginger, curry powder, and cook for 30 seconds over low heat, stirring constantly. Stir in the pumpkin, broth, and salt to taste and bring to a boil. Reduce heat to low, cover, and simmer, uncovered, until the flavors are blended, about 15 minutes.

2. Use an immersion blender to puree the soup in the pot or transfer in batches to a blender or food processor, puree, then return to the pot, and season with salt and pepper to taste. Add coconut milk and heat until hot.

3. Ladle into soup bowls, sprinkle with parsley and a spoonful of chutney sprinkled with chopped cashews, if using, and serve.

Tofu and Spinach Lasagna with Red Sauce

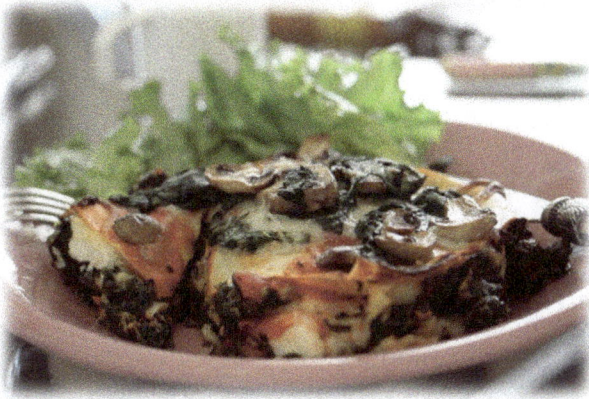

Preparation time: 20minutes

Cooking time: 45minutes

Serving: 4

Nutritional Values (Per Serving):

- Calories: 487
- Total Fat:45.3g

- Saturated Fat:34.2g
- Total Carbs: 13g
- Dietary Fiber:3g
- Sugar: 2g
- Protein: 14g
- Sodium:459 mg

Ingredients:

- 2 tbsp butter
- 1 white onion, chopped 1 garlic clove, minced
- 2 ½ cups crumbled tofu
- 3 tbsp tomato paste
- ½ tbsp dried oregano
- 1 tsp salt
- ¼ tsp ground black pepper
- ½ cup water
- 1 cup baby spinach

For the low-carb pasta:

- Flax egg: 8 tbsp flax seed powder + 1 ½ cups water
- 1 ½ cup dairy-free cashew cream
- 1 tsp salt

- 5 tbsp psyllium husk powder

For topping:

- 2 cups coconut cream
- 5 oz. shredded mozzarella cheese
- 2 oz. grated tofu cheese
- ½ tsp salt
- ¼ tsp ground black pepper
- ½ cup fresh parsley, finely chopped

Directions:

1. Melt the butter in a medium pot over medium heat. Then, add the white onion and garlic, and sauté until fragrant and soft, about 3 minutes.
2. Stir in the tofu and cook until brown. Mix in the tomato paste, oregano, salt, and black pepper.
3. Pour the water into the pot, stir, and simmer the ingredients until most of the liquid has evaporated.
4. While cooking the sauce, make the lasagna sheets. Preheat the oven to 300 F and mix the flax seed powder with the water in a medium bowl to make flax egg. Allow sitting to thicken for 5 minutes.

5. Combine the flax egg with the cashew cream and salt. Add the psyllium husk powder a bit at a time while whisking and allow the mixture to sit for a few more minutes.

6. Line a baking sheet with parchment paper and spread the mixture in. Cover with another parchment paper and use a rolling pin to flatten the dough into the sheet.

7. Bake the batter in the oven for 10 to 12 minutes, remove after, take off the parchment papers, and slice the pasta into sheets that fit your baking dish.

8. In a bowl, combine the coconut cream and two-thirds of the mozzarella cheese. Fetch out 2 tablespoons of the mixture and reserve.

9. Mix in the tofu cheese, salt, black pepper, and parsley. Set aside.

10. Grease your baking dish with cooking spray and lay in one-third of the pasta sheet; spread half of the tomato sauce on top, add another one-third set of the pasta sheets, the remaining tomato sauce and the rest of the pasta sheets.

11. Grease your baking dish with cooking spray, layer a single line of pasta in the dish, spread with some tomato sauce, 1/3 of the spinach, and ¼ of the coconut cream mixture. Season with salt and black pepper as desired.

12. Repeat layering the ingredients twice in the same manner making sure to top the final layer with the coconut cream mixture and the reserved cashew cream.
13. Bake in the oven for 30 minutes at 400 F or until the lasagna has a beautiful
14. brown surface.
15. Remove the dish; allow cooling for a few minutes, and slice.
16. Serve the lasagna with a baby green salad.

Zoodle Bolognese

Preparation time: 10minutes

Cooking time: 35minutes

Serving: 4

Nutritional Values (Per Serving):

- Calories: ,23
- Total Fat:14.7g
- Saturated Fat:8.1g
- Total Carbs: 14g
- Dietary Fiber:1g
- Sugar:7 g
- Protein: 13g
- Sodium: 530mg

Ingredients:

For the Bolognese sauce:

- 3 oz. olive oil
- 1 white onion, chopped

- 1 garlic clove, minced
- 3 oz. celery, chopped
- 3 cups crumbled tofu
- 2 tbsp tomato paste
- 1 ½ cups crushed tomatoes
- 1 tsp salt
- ¼ tsp black pepper
- 1 tbsp dried basil
- 1 tbsp Worcestershire sauce
- Water as needed

For the zoodles:

- 1 lb zucchinis
- 2 tbsp butter
- Salt and black pepper to taste

Directions:

1. Pour the olive oil into a saucepan and heat over medium heat. When no longer shimmering, add the onion, garlic, and celery. Sauté for 3 minutes or until the onions are soft and the carrots caramelized.

2. Pour in the tofu, tomato paste, tomatoes, salt, black pepper, basil, and Worcestershire sauce. Stir and cook for 15 minutes, or simmer for 30 minutes.

3. Mix in some water if the mixture is too thick and simmer further for 20 minutes.

4. While the sauce cooks, make the zoodles. Run the zucchini through a spiralizer to form noodles.

5. Melt the butter in a skillet over medium heat and toss the zoodles quickly in the butter, about 1 minute only.

6. Season with salt and black pepper.

Indonesian Green Bean Salad with Cabbage and Carrots

Preparation time: 15 minutes

Cooking time: 0 minutes

Servings: 4

Ingredients:

- 2 cups green beans, trimmed and cut into 1-inch pieces
- 2 medium carrots, cut into 1/4-inch slices
- 2 cups finely shredded cabbage
- 1/3 cup golden raisins
- 1/4 cup unsalted roasted peanuts
- 1 garlic clove, minced
- 1 medium shallot, chopped
- 11/2 teaspoons grated fresh ginger
- 1/3 cup creamy peanut butter
- 2 tablespoons soy sauce

- 2 tablespoons fresh lemon juice
- 1 teaspoon sugar (optional)
- 1/4 teaspoon salt (optional)
- 1/8 teaspoon ground cayenne
- 3/4 cup unsweetened coconut milk

Directions:

1 Lightly steam the green beans, carrots, and cabbage for about 5 minutes, then place them in a large bowl. Add the raisins and peanuts and set aside to cool.

2 In a food processor or blender, puree the garlic, shallot, and ginger. Add the peanut butter, soy sauce, lemon juice, sugar, salt, and cayenne, and process until blended. Add the coconut milk and blend until smooth. Pour the dressing over the salad, toss gently to combine, and serve.

Cucumber and Onion Quinoa Salad

Preparation time: 15 minutes

Cooking time: 20 minutes

Servings: 4

Nutritional Values (Per Serving):

- Calories: 369
- Fat: 11g
- Protein: 10g
- Carbohydrates: 58g
- Fiber: 6g
- Sugar: 12g
- Sodium: 88mg

Ingredients:

- 1½ cups dry quinoa, rinsed and drained

- 2¼ cups water
- ⅓ cup white wine vinegar
- 2tablespoons extra-virgin olive oil
- 1 tablespoon chopped fresh dill
- 1½ teaspoons vegan sugar
- 2 pinches salt
- ¼ teaspoon freshly ground black pepper
- 2 cups sliced sweet onions
- 2 cups diced cucumber
- 4 cups shredded lettuce

Directions:

1. In a medium pot, combine the quinoa and water. Bring to a boil.
2. Cover, reduce the heat to medium-low, and simmer for 15 to 20 minutes, until the water is absorbed. Remove from the stove and let stand for 5 minutes. Fluff with a fork and set aside.
3. Meanwhile, in a small bowl, mix the vinegar, olive oil, dill, sugar, salt, and pepper. Set aside. Into each of 4 wide-mouth jars, add 2 tablespoons of dressing, ½ cup of onions, ½ cup of cucumber, 1 cup of cooked quinoa, and 1 cup of shredded lettuce. Seal the lids tightly.

Moroccan Aubergine Salad

Preparation time: 30 minutes

Cooking time: 15 minutes

Servings: 2

Nutrition:

- Calories: 97
- Total fat: 4g
- Carbs: 16g
- Fiber: 8g
- Protein: 4g

Ingredients:

- 1 teaspoon olive oil
- 1 eggplant, diced
- ½ teaspoon ground cumin
- ½ teaspoon ground ginger
- ¼ teaspoon turmeric

- ¼ teaspoon ground nutmeg
- Pinch sea salt
- 1 lemon, half zested and juiced, half cut into wedges
- 2 tablespoons capers
- 1 tablespoon chopped green olives
- 1 garlic clove, pressed
- Handful fresh mint, finely chopped
- 2 cups spinach, chopped

Directions:

1. Heat the oil in a large skillet on medium heat, then sauté the eggplant. Once it has softened slightly, about 5 minutes, stir in the cumin, ginger, turmeric, nutmeg, and salt. Cook until the eggplant is very soft, about 10 minutes.

2. Add the lemon zest and juice, capers, olives, garlic, and mint. Sauté for another minute or two, to blend the flavors. Put a handful of spinach on each plate, and spoon the eggplant mixture on top.

3. Serve with a wedge of lemon, to squeeze the fresh juice over the greens.

4. To tenderize the eggplant and reduce some of its naturally occurring bitter taste, you can sweat the

eggplant by salting it. After dicing the eggplant, sprinkle it with salt and let it sit in a colander for about 30 minutes. Rinse the eggplant to remove the salt, then continue with the recipe as written.

Potato Salad with Artichoke Hearts

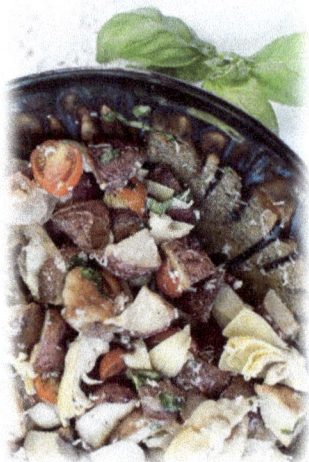

Preparation time: 15 minutes

Cooking time: 15 minutes

Servings: 4 to 6

Ingredients:

- 1½ pounds Yukon Gold potatoes, peeled and cut into 1-inch dice

- 1 (10-ouncepackage frozen artichoke hearts, cooked
- 2 cups halved ripe grape tomatoes
- 1⁄2 cup frozen peas, thawed
- 3 green onions, minced
- 1 tablespoon minced fresh parsley
- 1⁄3 cup olive oil
- 2 tablespoons fresh lemon juice
- 1 garlic clove, minced
- Salt and freshly ground black pepper

Directions:

1. In a large pot of boiling salted water, cook the potatoes until just tender but still firm, about 15 minutes. Drain well and transfer to a large bowl.
2. Quarter the artichokes and add them to the potatoes. Add the tomatoes, peas, green onions, and parsley and set aside.
3. In a small bowl, combine the oil, lemon juice, garlic, and salt and pepper to taste. Mix well, pour the dressing over potato salad, and toss gently to combine. Set aside at room temperature to allow flavors to blend, about 20 minutes. Taste, adjusting seasonings if necessary, and serve.

Capers Dip

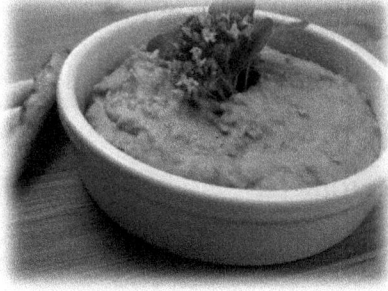

Preparation time: 10 minutes

Cooking time: 20 minutes

Servings: 4

Nutritional Values (Per Serving):

- Calories 127
- Fat 3
- Fiber 3
- Carbs 6
- Protein 7

Ingredients:

- 2 tablespoons olive oil
- 4 scallions, chopped
- 1 teaspoon rosemary, dried
- 2 tablespoons capers, drained
- 1 cup coconut cream
- 2 tablespoons pine nuts
- 1 bunch basil, chopped

Directions:

1. Heat up a pan with the oil over medium heat, add the scallions and the capers and sauté for 5 minutes.
2. Add the cream and the other ingredients, stir, cook over medium heat for 15 minutes more, blend using an immersion blender, divide into bowls and serve.

Radish and Walnuts Dip

Preparation time: 10 minutes

Cooking time: 20 minutes

Servings: 4

Nutritional Values (Per Serving):

- Calories 192
- Fat 5
- Fiber 7
- Carbs 12
- Protein 5

Ingredients:

- 2 tablespoons walnuts, chopped
- 1 cup coconut cream
- 2 cups radishes, chopped
- 4 scallions, chopped
- 2 tablespoons olive oil

- 1 teaspoon chili powder
- A pinch of salt and black pepper
- 2 teaspoons mustard powder
- 2 teaspoons garlic powder
- 2 teaspoons cumin, ground

Directions:

1. Heat up a pan with the oil over medium heat, add the scallions, mustard powder, garlic powder and cumin, stir and sauté for 5 minutes.
2. Add the walnuts, and the otheringredients, stir, cook over medium heat for 15 minutes, blend well using an immersion blender, divide into bowls and serve.

Mushroom Cakes

Preparation time: 10 minutes

Cooking time: 12 minutes

Servings: 6

Nutritional Values (Per Serving):

- calories 222
- fat 4
- fiber 3
- carbs 8
- protein 10

Ingredients:

- 1 cup shallots, chopped
- 2 tablespoons olive oil
- 3 garlic cloves, minced
- 1 pound mushrooms, minced
- 2 tablespoons almond flour

- ¼ cup coconut cream
- 1 tablespoon flaxseed mixed with 2 tablespoons water
- ¼ cup parsley, chopped

Directions:

1. In a bowl, combine the shallots with the garlic, the mushrooms and the otheringredients except the oil, stir well and shape medium cakes out of this mix.
2. Heat up a pan with the oil over medium heat, add the mushroom cakes, cook for 6 minutes on each side, arrange them on a platter and serve as an appetizer.

Cabbage Sticks

Preparation time: 10 minutes

Cooking time: 30 minutes

Servings: 4

Nutritional Values (Per Serving):

- Calories 300
- Fat 4
- Fiber 7
- Carbs 18
- Protein 6

Ingredients:

- 1 pound cabbage, leaves separated and cut into thick strips
- 1 tablespoon olive oil
- 1 tablespoon balsamic vinegar
- 1 teaspoon ginger, grated

- 1 teaspoon hot paprika
- A pinch of salt and black pepper

Directions:

1. Spread the cabbage strips on a baking sheet lined with parchment paper, add the oil, the vinegar and the otheringredients, toss and cook at 400 degrees F for 30 minutes.
2. Divide the cabbage strips into bowls and serve as a snack.

Crispy Brussels Sprouts

Preparation time: 10 minutes

Cooking time: 30 minutes

Servings: 4

Nutritional Values (Per Serving):

- Calories 162
- Fat 4
- Fiber 3
- Carbs 7
- Protein 8

Ingredients:

- 2 pounds Brussels sprouts, trimmed and halved
- 1 teaspoon red pepper flakes
- 1 tablespoon smoked paprika
- 2 tablespoons avocado oil

- 1 tablespoon balsamic vinegar
- A pinch of salt and black pepper

Directions:

1. In a roasting pan, combine the sprouts with the pepper flakes, paprika and the otheringredients, toss and cook at 400 degrees F for 30 minutes.
2. Divide the Brussels sprouts into bowls and serve as a snack.

Coconut Chocolate Cake

Preparation time: 10 minutes

Cooking time: 30 minutes

Servings: 12

Nutritional Values (Per Serving):

- Calories 268
- Fat 23.9
- Fiber 5.1
- Carbs 9.4
- Protein 6.1

Ingredients:

- 4 tablespoons flaxseed mixed with 5 tablespoons water
- 1 cup coconut flesh, unsweetened and shredded
- 1 teaspoon vanilla extract

- 2 tablespoons cocoa powder
- 1 teaspoon baking soda
- 2 cups almond flour
- 4 tablespoons stevia
- 2 tablespoons lime zest
- 2 cups coconut cream

Directions:

1. In a bowl, combine the flaxmeal with the coconut, the vanilla and the other ingredients, whisk well and transfer to a cake pan.
2. Cook the cake at 360 degrees F for 30 minutes, cool down and serve.

Mint Chocolate Cream

Preparation time: 10 minutes

Cooking time: 0 minutes

Servings: 6

Nutritional Values (Per Serving):

- Calories 514
- Fat 56
- Fiber 3.9
- Carbs 7.8
- Protein 3

Ingredients:

- 1 cup coconut oil, melted
- 4 tablespoons cocoa powder
- 1 teaspoon vanilla extract
- 1 cup mint, chopped

- 2 cups coconut cream

- 4 tablespoons stevia

Directions:

1. In your food processor, combine the coconut oil with the cocoa powder, the cream and the other ingredients, pulse well, divide into bowls and serve really cold.

Cranberries Cake

Preparation time: 10 minutes

Cooking time: 30 minutes

Servings: 6

Nutritional Values (Per Serving):

- Calories 244
- Fat 16.7
- Fiber 11.8
- Carbs 21.3
- Protein 4.4

Ingredients:

- 2 cups coconut flour
- 2 tablespoon coconut oil, melted
- 3 tablespoons stevia
- 1 tablespoon cocoa powder, unsweetened
- 2 tablespoons flaxseed mixed with 3 tablespoons water

- 1 cup cranberries
- 1 cup coconut cream
- ¼ teaspoon vanilla extract
- ½ teaspoon baking powder

Directions:

1. In a bowl, combine the coconut flour with the coconut oil, the stevia and the other ingredients, and whisk well.
2. Pour this into a cake pan lined with parchment paper, introduce in the oven and cook at 360 degrees F for 30 minutes.
3. Cool down, slice and serve.

Sweet Zucchini Buns

Preparation time: 10 minutes

Cooking time: 30 minutes

Servings: 8

Nutritional Values (Per Serving):

- Calories 169
- Fat 15.3
- Fiber 3.9
- Carbs 6.4
- Protein 3.2

Ingredients:

- 1 cup almond flour
- 1/3 cup coconut flesh, unsweetened and shredded
- 1 cup zucchinis, grated
- 2 tablespoons stevia
- 1 teaspoon baking soda

- ½ teaspoon cinnamon powder
- 3 tablespoons flaxseed mixed with 4 tablespoons water
- 1 cup coconut cream

Directions:

1. In a bowl, mix the almond flour with the coconut flesh, the zucchinis and the other ingredients, stir well until you obtain a dough, shape 8 buns and arrange them on a baking sheet lined with parchment paper.
2. Introduce in the oven at 350 degrees and bake for 30 minutes.
3. Serve these sweet buns warm.

Lime Custard

Preparation time: 10 minutes

Cooking time: 20 minutes

Servings: 6

Nutritional Values (Per Serving):

- Calories 234
- Fat 21.6
- Fiber 4.3
- Carbs 9
- Protein 3.5

Ingredients:

- 1 pint almond milk
- 4 tablespoons lime zest, grated
- 3 tablespoons lime juice
- 3 tablespoons flaxseed mixed with 4 tablespoons water

- 2 tablespoons stevia
- 2 teaspoons vanilla extract

Directions:

1. In a bowl, combine the almond milk with the lime zest, lime juice and the other ingredients, whisk well and divide into 4 ramekins.
2. Bake in the oven at 360 degrees F for 30 minutes.
3. Cool the custard down and serve.

Warm Rum Butter Spiced Cider

Preparation time: 15 Minutes

Servings: 4

Ingredients:

- 3/4 cup rum
- 4 cups apple cider
- 2 cinnamon sticks
- 4 cardamom pods
- 1/4 teaspoon ground allspice
- 4 whole cloves
- 1 teaspoon lime juice
- 4 teaspoons nondairy butter

Directions:

1. Combine all the ingredients in the instant pot. Seal the lid and cook on high 5 minutes. Let the pressure release naturally.

Peppermint Patty Cocoa

Preparation time: 15 Minutes

Servings: 4

Ingredients:

- 4 cups almond milk
- 3 ounces semisweet chocolate chips
- 1 teaspoon cocoa powder
- 1 teaspoon vanilla extract
- 1/4 cup sugar
- 1 tablespoon agave nectar
- 1 teaspoon peppermint extract

Directions:

1. Combine all the ingreidients in the instant pot. Seal the lid and cook on high 4 minutes, then let the pressure release naturally.
2. Serve garnished with a sprig of mint or topped with vegan marshmallows!

Apple & Walnut Cake

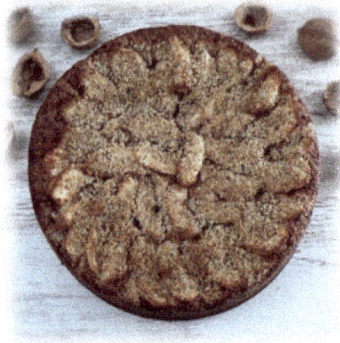

Preparation time: 20 Minutes

Servings: 6

Ingredients:

- 1¾ cups unbleached all-purpose flour
- 1 cup unsweetened applesauce
- ⅔ cup packed light brown sugar
- ½ cup chopped walnuts
- ¼ cup vegetable oil
- 1 tablespoon freshly squeezed lemon juice
- 1 teaspoon pure vanilla extract
- 1½ teaspoons ground cinnamon
- 1 teaspoon baking powder
- ½ teaspoon baking soda

- ½ teaspoon salt
- ¼ teaspoon ground allspice
- ¼ teaspoon ground nutmeg
- ⅛ teaspoon ground cloves

Directions:

1. Lightly oil a baking tray that will fit in the steamer basket of your Instant Pot.
2. In a bowl, combine the flour, baking powder, baking soda, sugar, cinnamon, allspice, nutmeg, cloves, and salt.
3. In another bowl combine the applesauce, oil, vanilla, and lemon juice.
4. Stir the wet mixture into the dry mixture slowly until they form a smooth mix.
5. Fold in the walnuts.
6. Pour the batter into your baking tray and put the tray in your steamer basket.
7. Pour the minimum amount of water into the base of your Instant Pot and lower the steamer basket.
8. Seal and cook on Steam for 12 minutes.
9. Release the pressure quickly and set to one side to cool a little.

Lemon Garlic Mushrooms

Preparation time: 10 minutes

Cooking time: 15 minutes

Servings: 4

Nutritions:

- Calories 87
- Fat 5.6 g
- Carbohydrates 7.5 g
- Sugar 1.8 g
- Protein 3 g
- Cholesterol 8 mg

Ingredients:

- 3 oz enoki mushrooms
- 1 tbsp olive oil

- 1 tsp lemon zest, chopped
- 2 tbsp lemon juice
- 3 garlic cloves, sliced
- 6 oyster mushrooms, halved
- 5 oz cremini mushrooms, sliced
- 1/2 red chili, sliced
- 1/2 onion, sliced
- 1 tsp sea salt

Directions:

1. Heat olive oil in a pan over high heat.
2. Add shallots, enoki mushrooms, oyster mushrooms, cremini mushrooms, and chili.
3. Stir well and cook over medium-high heat for 10 minutes.
4. Add lemon zest and stir well. Season with lemon juice and salt and cook for 3-4 minutes.
5. Serve and enjoy.

Almond Green Beans

Preparation time: 10 minutes

Cooking time: 10 minutes

Servings: 4

Nutritions:

- Calories 146
- Fat 11.2 g
- Carbohydrates 10.9 g
- Sugar 2 g
- Protein 4 g
- Cholesterol 0 mg

Ingredients:

- 1 lb fresh green beans, trimmed
- 1/3 cup almonds, sliced
- 4 garlic cloves, sliced
- 2 tbsp olive oil

- 1 tbsp lemon juice
- ½ tsp sea salt

Directions:

1. Add green beans, salt, and lemon juice in a mixing bowl. Toss well and set aside.
2. Heat oil in a pan over medium heat.
3. Add sliced almonds and sauté until lightly browned.
4. Add garlic and sauté for 30 seconds.
5. Pour almond mixture over green beans and toss well.
6. Stir well and serve immediately.

Fried Okra

Preparation time: 10 minutes

Cooking time: 10 minutes

Servings: 4

Nutritions:

- Calories 91
- Fat 4.2 g
- Carbohydrates 10.2 g
- Sugar 10.2 g
- Protein 3.9 g
- Cholesterol 0 mg

Ingredients:

- 1 lb fresh okra, cut into ¼" slices
- 1/3 cup almond meal
- Pepper Salt
- Oil for frying

Directions:

1. Heat oil in large pan over medium-high heat.
2. In a bowl, mix together sliced okra, almond meal, pepper, and salt until well coated.
3. Once the oil is hot then add okra to the hot oil and cook until lightly browned.
4. Remove fried okra from pan and allow to drain on paper towels.
5. Serve and enjoy.

Tomato Avocado Cucumber Salad

Preparation time: 10 minutes

Cooking time: 0 minutes

Serves: 4

Nutritions:

- Calories 130
- Fat 9.8 g
- Carbohydrates 10.6 g
- Sugar 5.1 g
- Protein 2.1 g
- Cholesterol 0 mg

Ingredients:

- 1 cucumber, sliced avocado, chopped
- ½ onion, sliced tomatoes, chopped

- 1 bell pepper, chopped
- ¼ tsp garlic powder tbsp olive oil
- 1 tbsp lemon juice
- ½ tsp black pepper
- ½ tsp salt

For Dressings:

- 1 tbsp cilantro

Directions:

1. In a small bowl, mix together all dressing ingredients and set aside.
2. Add all salad ingredients into the large mixing bowl and mix well.
3. Pour dressing over salad and toss well.
4. Serve immediately and enjoy.

Asian Cucumber Salad

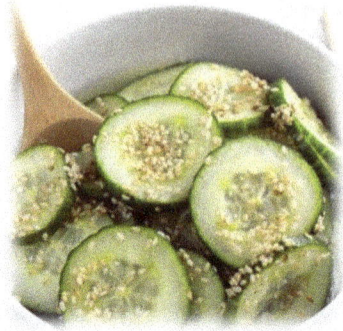

Preparation time: 10 minutes

Cooking time: 0 minutes

Servings: 6

Nutritions:

- Calories 27
- Fat 0.7 g
- Carbohydrates 3.5 g
- Sugar 1.6 g
- Protein 0.7 g
- Cholesterol 0 mg

Ingredients:

- 4 cups cucumbers, sliced
- ¼ tsp red pepper flakes
- ½ tsp sesame oil
- 1 tsp sesame seeds
- ¼ cup rice wine vinegar
- ¼ cup red pepper, diced
- ¼ cup onion, sliced
- ½ tsp sea salt

Directions:

1. Add all ingredients into the mixing bowl and toss well.
2. Serve immediately and enjoy.

Roasted Carrots

Preparation time: 10 minutes

Cooking time: 35 minutes

Servings: 6

Nutritions:

- Calories 139
- Fat 9.4 g
- Carbohydrates 14.2 g
- Sugar 6.6 g
- Protein 1.3 g
- Cholesterol 0 mg

Ingredients:

- 16 small carrots
- 1 tbsp fresh parsley, chopped
- 1 tbsp dried basil
- 6 garlic cloves, minced

- 4 tbsp olive oil
- 1 1/2 tsp salt

Directions:

1. Preheat the oven to 375 F/ 190 C.
2. In a bowl, combine together oil, carrots, basil, garlic, and salt.
3. Spread the carrots onto a baking tray and bake in preheated oven for 35 minutes.
4. Garnish with parsley and serve.

www.ingramcontent.com/pod-product-compliance
Lightning Source LLC
Chambersburg PA
CBHW050747030426
42336CB00012B/1700